THE CASTOR OIL BIBLE

The Complete Guide To Transform Your Health And Beauty With The Power Of Castor Oil

Mercci Jordan

TABLE OF CONTENTS

THE CASTOR OIL BIBLE I

THE HISTORY OF CASTOR OIL 6

UNDERSTANDING CASTOR OIL 16

- WHAT IS CASTOR OIL? 16
- CHEMICAL COMPOSITION OF CASTOR OIL 18
- PHYSICAL AND THERAPEUTIC PROPERTIES 19
- TYPES OF CASTOR OIL (COLD-PRESSED VS. REFINED VS. BLACK CASTOR OIL) 20

CASTOR OIL AND HEALTH BENEFITS 28

- ANTI-INFLAMMATORY AND PAIN RELIEF PROPERTIES 28
- HOW CASTOR OIL HELPS WITH PAIN AND INFLAMMATION: 29
- BOOSTING IMMUNITY AND DETOXIFYING THE BODY 30
- HOW CASTOR OIL SUPPORTS IMMUNITY AND DETOXIFICATION: 31
- SUPPORTING DIGESTIVE HEALTH (CONSTIPATION, GUT HEALING) 32
- HOW CASTOR OIL SUPPORTS DIGESTION: 33
- IMPROVING LYMPHATIC DRAINAGE AND CIRCULATION 34
- HOW CASTOR OIL HELPS WITH CIRCULATION & LYMPH FLOW: 35

CASTOR OIL FOR SKIN AND BEAUTY 39

- NATURAL MOISTURIZER FOR DRY SKIN 40
- HOW CASTOR OIL HELPS WITH SKIN CONDITIONS: 42
- ANTI-AGING PROPERTIES (REDUCING WRINKLES AND FINE LINES) 44
- WHY CASTOR OIL IS GREAT FOR ANTI-AGING: 44
- TREATING SCARS, STRETCH MARKS, AND BLEMISHES 45

CASTOR OIL FOR HAIR AND SCALP HEALTH 50

- STIMULATING HAIR GROWTH AND PREVENTING HAIR LOSS 50
- HOW CASTOR OIL HELPS WITH HAIR GROWTH: 51

CASTOR OIL FOR EYE AND ORAL HEALTH 61

Reducing Dark Circles and Puffy Eyes 62

CASTOR OIL FOR JOINT AND MUSCLE PAIN 71

Using Castor Oil for Arthritis and Joint Pain Relief 71

CASTOR OIL AND WOMEN'S HEALTH 79

Balancing Menstrual Cycles and Reducing PMS Symptoms 80

Fertility and Castor Oil (Enhancing Reproductive Health) 82

CASTOR OIL FOR DETOX AND INTERNAL HEALING 89

Liver Cleansing and Detoxification 90

CASTOR OIL FOR BABIES AND KIDS 99

Treating Colic and Constipation in Infants 100

How Castor Oil Helps with Cough Relief: 105

CASTOR OIL FOR PETS AND ANIMALS 107

Castor Oil for Wound Healing in Dogs and Cats 108

How Castor Oil Helps with Wound Healing: 108

CASTOR OIL FOR HOME AND EVERYDAY USES 116

Natural Wood Polish and Leather Conditioner 116

Castor Oil for Lubricating Machinery and Tools 119

How Castor Oil Works as a Lubricant: 119

DIY CASTOR OIL RECIPES AND REMEDIES 127

Homemade Castor Oil Hair Growth Serum 127

Healing Castor Oil Face Cream 129

Castor Oil Massage Blend for Pain Relief 133

Ingredients: 133

CONCLUSION 137

Where to Buy High-Quality Castor Oil 141

Recommended Sources for Buying Castor Oil: 142

FREQUENTLY ASKED QUESTIONS (FAQS) 144

The History of Castor Oil

Castor oil has a rich and fascinating history that spans thousands of years, touching various civilizations, medical traditions, and modern scientific research. This chapter explores how castor oil has been revered for its healing properties since ancient times and how its uses have evolved into modern medicine.

Ancient Civilizations and Castor Oil (Egypt, India, Greece)

Ancient Egypt: The Oil of Pharaohs

Castor oil was highly valued in ancient Egypt, where it was known as a **miracle elixir** for beauty, medicine, and daily life. Archaeologists have discovered **castor beans in tombs dating back to 4000 BC**, proving its importance in Egyptian culture.

- **Beauty & Skincare** – Egyptian women, including Queen Cleopatra, reportedly used castor oil to **moisturize their skin, lengthen eyelashes, and promote hair growth**.
- **Medicinal Uses** – Egyptian healers prescribed castor oil as a remedy for **constipation, eye infections, and wound healing**.

- **Lamp Fuel** – The oil was also used as fuel for **lamps**, providing a steady source of light in homes and temples.

India: Ayurveda and the Healing Power of Castor Oil

In **Ayurvedic medicine**, castor oil (known as ERANDA TAILA) has been used for over **3,000 years** as a **therapeutic oil**. The **Ayurvedic texts** describe castor oil as having **warming, detoxifying, and pain-relieving** properties.

- Used in **Panchakarma therapy** (Ayurvedic detox) to remove toxins from the body.

- Applied externally to treat **joint pain, inflammation, and skin conditions**.
- Ingested to **relieve constipation** and promote digestive health.
- Used in postnatal care to aid in **recovery after childbirth**.

Ancient Greece: The Physician's Choice

The famous Greek physician **Hippocrates (c. 460–370 BC)**, often called the **Father of Medicine**, documented the use of castor oil for:

- **Digestive disorders** – As a natural laxative and cleanser.
- **Skin conditions** – Healing **wounds, burns, and infections**.

- **Pain relief** – Treating **muscle and joint pain**.

The Greek and Roman civilizations embraced castor oil, spreading its use across Europe and influencing early Western medicine.

Castor Oil in Traditional Medicine

As castor oil spread across continents, it became a cornerstone of **traditional medicine** in many cultures.

- **Traditional Chinese Medicine (TCM)** – Used for its **anti-inflammatory and detoxifying** properties, often applied to ease **joint pain and swelling**.

- **African Traditional Medicine** – Used for **wound healing, skin infections, and digestive issues**.
- **Native American Remedies** – Indigenous tribes in North America used castor oil as a **natural remedy for colds, constipation, and muscle pain**.
- **European Folk Medicine** – Herbalists in medieval Europe recommended castor oil for **treating infections, promoting hair growth, and soothing sore muscles**.

Castor oil remained a household remedy in many cultures well into the 19th and 20th centuries.

The Role of Castor Oil in Modern Science and Medicine

With advancements in modern medicine, **scientific research** has confirmed many of the traditional uses of castor oil. Today, it is recognized for its **unique composition** and **therapeutic benefits** in several medical fields.

Key Scientific Discoveries About Castor Oil

- **Ricinoleic Acid** – Castor oil is rich in **ricinoleic acid (up to 90%)**, a rare fatty acid responsible for its **anti-inflammatory, antimicrobial, and pain-relieving properties**.
- **Lymphatic and Immune Support** – Research shows that **castor oil packs**

stimulate the **lymphatic system**, enhancing detoxification and immune function.

- **Antimicrobial Properties** – Studies confirm that castor oil has natural **antibacterial and antifungal** effects, making it useful for **wound care and skin infections**.
- **Hair Growth and Skin Health** – The oil's ability to **moisturize, repair damaged skin, and promote hair growth** has been backed by dermatological research.

Modern Medical Uses of Castor Oil

- **Pharmaceuticals** – Used as an ingredient in **medications, including laxatives, pain relief creams, and eye drops**.

- **Surgical Applications** – Castor oil derivatives are used in making **biodegradable medical implants and coatings for drug delivery systems**.
- **Cancer Research** – Some studies suggest that castor oil compounds can be used in **targeted drug delivery for chemotherapy**.
- **Cosmetic and Skincare Industry** – Found in **natural moisturizers, anti-aging creams, and hair growth serums**.

Castor Oil in Alternative Medicine

- **Holistic Healing & Detoxification** – Naturopaths and wellness practitioners recommend **castor oil packs** for **liver detox, hormone balance, and pain relief**.

- **Aromatherapy & Massage Therapy** – Used in **carrier oils and therapeutic massages** for relaxation and healing.

Understanding Castor Oil

Castor oil is a unique and powerful natural remedy that has been used for centuries for its wide range of health, beauty, and industrial benefits. To fully appreciate its potential, it's essential to understand its composition, extraction methods, different types, and how to select the highest-quality oil for your needs.

What is Castor Oil?

Ricinus communis plant, commonly known as the **castor bean plant**. The extraction process determines the oil's purity, potency, and overall effectiveness.

1. **Harvesting** – The seeds of the castor plant are harvested and dried.
2. **Shell Removal** – The outer shell is removed to extract the inner castor bean.
3. **Oil Extraction Methods:**
    - **Cold-Pressing:** The beans are mechanically pressed without heat to retain the highest level of nutrients.
    - **Solvent Extraction:** Chemical solvents (like hexane) are used to extract more oil but may reduce purity.
    - **Boiling (Traditional Method):** Beans are boiled, and the oil rises to the surface, which is then collected.

Chemical Composition of Castor Oil

Castor oil is unique among vegetable oils due to its high concentration of **ricinoleic acid**—a rare fatty acid that gives the oil its powerful healing properties.

- **Ricinoleic Acid (85-90%)** – Anti-inflammatory, antibacterial, antifungal, and deeply moisturizing.
- **Oleic Acid (2-6%)** – Helps with skin hydration and hair conditioning.
- **Linoleic Acid (1-5%)** – An omega-6 fatty acid that supports skin regeneration.
- **Stearic Acid (0.5-1%)** – Adds thickness and creaminess, beneficial for skincare products.

- **Vitamin E** – Acts as an antioxidant, protecting skin from damage.

Physical and Therapeutic Properties

- **Color** – Pale yellow to clear (except Jamaican Black Castor Oil, which is dark brown/black).
- **Texture** – Thick, sticky, and highly viscous.
- **Smell** – Mild, nutty scent (stronger in roasted varieties like Jamaican Black Castor Oil).
- **Taste** – Slightly bitter, but commonly used in small medicinal doses.
- **Absorption** – Slow absorption rate, making it ideal for deep penetration in skin and hair treatments.

Types of Castor Oil (Cold-Pressed vs. Refined vs. Black Castor Oil)

There are several types of castor oil, each with distinct characteristics and uses. Choosing the right one depends on your specific needs.

1. Cold-Pressed Castor Oil (Virgin Castor Oil)

✅ **Extraction:** Pressed from raw castor beans without heat, preserving nutrients.

✅ **Color:** Pale yellow, light golden.

✅ **Texture:** Thick and smooth.

✅ **Nutritional Value: Highest concentration of ricinoleic acid**, retaining full medicinal properties.

✅ **Best For:**

Skincare (acne, wrinkles, scars)

Hair growth and scalp health

Digestive health and detox

Natural anti-inflammatory and pain relief

❖ **Pros:** Purest form, no chemicals, best for medicinal and therapeutic use.

❖ **Cons:** More expensive than refined varieties.

2. Refined Castor Oil

✓ **Extraction:** Processed using heat or solvents to extract maximum oil.

✓ **Color:** Clear or very light yellow.

✓ **Texture:** Less thick than cold-pressed oil.

✓ **Nutritional Value:** Loses some nutrients due to

processing.

✓ **Best For:**

Industrial use (lubricants, coatings, cosmetics)

Less potent health remedies (laxative, minor skincare use)

◈ **Pros:** More affordable and available in large quantities.

◆ **Cons:** May contain fewer active compounds and might include additives.

3. Jamaican Black Castor Oil (JBCO)

✓ **Extraction:** Beans are roasted before pressing, giving the oil a darker color and stronger scent.

✓ **Color:** Dark brown to black.

✅ **Texture:** Thicker and heavier than cold-pressed castor oil.

✅ **Nutritional Value:** The roasting process enhances some nutrients but also removes certain delicate compounds.

✅ **Best For:**

Hair growth and thickening

Deep scalp conditioning and dandruff treatment

Pain relief and muscle relaxation

Eyelash and eyebrow enhancement

◈ **Pros:** Works exceptionally well for hair growth and scalp health.

◆ **Cons:** Has a strong burnt smell, may stain clothing or sheets.

Other Varieties

Hydrogenated Castor Oil (Castor Wax) – Used in cosmetics and industrial applications.

Castor Oil Blends – Sometimes mixed with coconut or almond oil for additional benefits.

How to Choose the Best Quality Castor Oil

When purchasing castor oil, **quality matters**. Low-quality castor oil may contain harmful chemicals, additives, or impurities that reduce its effectiveness. Here's what to look for:

1. Check the Label and Certification

✅ **Cold-Pressed or Virgin Castor Oil** – Ensures the oil is extracted without heat or chemicals.

✅ **100% Pure and Organic** – Look for **USDA Organic, ECOCERT, or similar certifications** to avoid pesticides.

✅ **Hexane-Free** – Hexane is a chemical solvent that can be toxic; **always choose hexane-free castor oil**.

✅ **No Additives or Fillers** – Some oils are diluted with mineral oils or other substances—avoid these!

2. Examine the Packaging

✅ **Dark Glass Bottles** – Protects the oil from light exposure, preserving its potency.

✅ **Airtight Seal** – Prevents contamination and oxidation.

✅ **Avoid Plastic Bottles** – Plastic can leach chemicals into the oil over time.

3. Smell and Texture Test

✅ **Mild Nutty or Earthy Scent** – A strong, unpleasant odor could indicate rancidity.

✅ **Thick and Viscous** – Should not feel too watery or greasy.

✅ **No Cloudiness or Sediment** – Pure castor oil is clear or slightly yellow, except for Jamaican Black Castor Oil.

4. Buy from Trusted Sources

✅ **Reputable Brands** – Choose brands with **positive customer reviews and transparency about sourcing**.

✅ **Organic Health Stores & Certified Online Retailers** – Avoid buying from unknown or unverified sellers.

✅**Check Expiry Date** – Fresh castor oil has a shelf life of **1-2 years** if stored properly.

Castor Oil and Health Benefits

Castor oil is widely recognized for its powerful therapeutic properties, making it a staple in natural medicine for centuries. From reducing inflammation and pain to supporting digestion, detoxification, and hormonal balance, its healing potential is vast. In this chapter, we explore the science-backed health benefits of castor oil and how to use it effectively.

Anti-Inflammatory and Pain Relief Properties

One of the most well-documented benefits of castor oil is its **strong anti-inflammatory** effect, primarily due to its high concentration of **ricinoleic acid**. This unique fatty acid has been shown to reduce swelling, soothe pain, and support the body's natural healing processes.

How Castor Oil Helps with Pain and Inflammation:

✅ **Relieves Joint Pain & Arthritis** – Castor oil penetrates deep into the skin and helps reduce **stiffness, swelling, and discomfort** in joints affected by arthritis, rheumatoid arthritis, and osteoarthritis.

✅ **Soothes Muscle Pain & Cramps** – A gentle castor oil massage can ease **muscle soreness, tension, and menstrual cramps**.

✅ **Heals Sprains & Injuries** – Speeds up **recovery from strains, sprains, and bruises** by improving circulation to the affected area.

✅ **Reduces Back Pain** – Applying a warm **castor oil pack** over the lower back provides natural relief for **chronic back pain and sciatica**.

🔷 **How to Use:**

- Massage **warm castor oil** onto sore joints and muscles.
- Apply a **castor oil pack** (cloth soaked in castor oil, covered with a warm compress) for **30-60 minutes** to enhance absorption and pain relief.

Boosting Immunity and Detoxifying the Body

Castor oil is a powerful **immune booster** that helps the body eliminate toxins and fight infections. Its **detoxifying** properties work by stimulating the

lymphatic system, which is essential for flushing out waste and toxins.

How Castor Oil Supports Immunity and Detoxification:

✅ **Stimulates White Blood Cells (WBCs)** – Research suggests that castor oil **increases lymphocyte production**, strengthening the body's ability to fight infections.

✅ **Removes Toxins & Improves Liver Function** – Castor oil stimulates the **liver and gallbladder**, supporting the body's natural detox pathways.

✅ **Combats Bacterial & Fungal Infections** – Castor oil's **antimicrobial properties** help fight off harmful bacteria, yeast, and fungi.

◆ **How to Use:**

- Apply a **castor oil pack over the liver area** (right side of the abdomen) for **45-60 minutes** to aid detoxification.
- Take **a teaspoon of cold-pressed castor oil** once a week for internal cleansing (consult a doctor before ingestion).

Supporting Digestive Health (Constipation, Gut Healing)

Castor oil is one of the oldest and most effective **natural laxatives**, helping to relieve constipation and promote a healthy digestive system.

How Castor Oil Supports Digestion:

✅ **Relieves Constipation Naturally** – Castor oil acts as a **stimulant laxative**, increasing bowel movement within **4-6 hours** after consumption.

✅ **Promotes Gut Healing** – It helps soothe and repair **inflammation in the intestines**, benefiting people with **IBS, leaky gut, and colitis**.

✅ **Eliminates Parasites** – Castor oil's purgative effect helps remove **harmful gut bacteria and parasites**.

🔹 **How to Use:**

- For **constipation relief**, take **1 teaspoon of castor oil on an empty stomach** (mix with juice if needed).

- For **gut healing**, massage warm castor oil onto the **abdomen** to reduce inflammation and promote digestion.

⚠️ **Caution:** Do not take castor oil internally for more than **3 consecutive days**, as it may cause dehydration or dependency.

Improving Lymphatic Drainage and Circulation

The **lymphatic system** is responsible for eliminating toxins and waste from the body. When the lymphatic system is sluggish, it can lead to **fatigue, swelling, infections, and chronic pain**. Castor oil is one of the best natural remedies to **stimulate lymphatic drainage and improve blood circulation**.

How Castor Oil Helps with Circulation & Lymph Flow:

✅ **Reduces Swelling & Edema** – Castor oil **improves lymphatic drainage**, helping to relieve **swollen ankles, puffy eyes, and fluid retention**.

✅ **Enhances Blood Circulation** – By reducing **blood stagnation**, castor oil can help people suffering from **cold hands and feet, varicose veins, and poor circulation**.

✅ **Strengthens the Immune System** – A healthy **lymphatic system** means **fewer infections, less inflammation, and better overall health**.

🔷 **How to Use:**

- Apply a **castor oil pack to the lower abdomen** to support lymphatic drainage.
- Massage castor oil **along swollen lymph nodes** (neck, armpits, groin) to promote detoxification.

Castor Oil and Hormonal Balance

Castor oil can play a **significant role in balancing hormones**, making it beneficial for **women's reproductive health, thyroid function, and adrenal support**.

How Castor Oil Supports Hormonal Balance:

✅ **Supports the Thyroid Gland** – Castor oil packs placed over the **thyroid (neck area)** may help **reduce inflammation and regulate thyroid**

function.

✅ **Balances Estrogen & Progesterone** – Castor oil supports hormone detoxification, benefiting women with **PCOS, irregular periods, and menopause symptoms**.

✅ **Enhances Fertility** – Castor oil increases **circulation to the ovaries and uterus**, making it useful for **fertility treatments and menstrual health**.

✅ **Relieves Menstrual Pain & PMS** – Applying warm castor oil on the abdomen can **ease period cramps and bloating**.

◆ How to Use:

- **For Thyroid Health:** Apply a **castor oil pack on the neck** for 30-60 minutes.
- **For Menstrual Relief:** Massage **warm castor oil over the lower abdomen** during your cycle.
- **For Fertility Support:** Use castor oil packs **3-4 times a week before ovulation** to improve uterine health.

Caution: Avoid using castor oil packs during pregnancy unless approved by a healthcare provider.

Castor Oil for Skin and Beauty

Castor oil is a **powerful natural remedy** for skin health, widely used in skincare routines for centuries. With its **rich fatty acid content, antibacterial properties, and deep moisturizing abilities**, castor oil can transform your skin, keeping it youthful, radiant, and problem-free.

This chapter explores **how castor oil benefits the skin**, how to use it for **common skin issues**, and easy **DIY treatments** you can incorporate into your beauty routine.

Natural Moisturizer for Dry Skin

Castor oil is an **excellent natural emollient**, deeply hydrating the skin while creating a protective barrier to prevent moisture loss. Unlike synthetic moisturizers, it **penetrates deep into the skin**, softening rough patches and **restoring hydration** without clogging pores.

Why Castor Oil Works as a Moisturizer:

✅ **Rich in Ricinoleic Acid** – A unique fatty acid that **locks in moisture** and protects against dryness.

✅ **Boosts Collagen Production** – Helps maintain **skin elasticity**, preventing **flakiness and rough patches**.

✅ **Soothes Itchy, Irritated Skin** – Perfect for **eczema, psoriasis, and sensitive skin** conditions.

🔷 **How to Use:**

- Apply **a few drops** of castor oil to clean, damp skin as a natural moisturizer.
- Mix **equal parts castor oil and coconut oil** for a lighter, more spreadable lotion.
- Use castor oil as a **nighttime facial oil** for deep hydration.

Pro Tip: If castor oil feels too thick, mix it with a lighter oil like **jojoba or almond oil**.

Healing Acne, Eczema, and Psoriasis

Thanks to its **antibacterial, antifungal, and anti-inflammatory** properties, castor oil is highly effective in treating **acne, eczema, and psoriasis**. It **reduces redness, soothes irritation, and promotes skin healing** without the harsh side effects of chemical treatments.

How Castor Oil Helps with Skin Conditions:

✅ **Acne** – Fights acne-causing bacteria, reduces breakouts, and prevents scarring.

✅ **Eczema & Psoriasis** – Hydrates dry, flaky patches while reducing itching and inflammation.

✅ **Fungal Skin Infections** – Treats ringworm, athlete's foot, and scalp infections.

How to Use for Acne:

- Apply **a drop of castor oil** directly on pimples as an overnight spot treatment.
- Mix with **tea tree oil** for extra antibacterial power.

How to Use for Eczema/Psoriasis:

- Warm castor oil and gently massage onto affected areas **twice daily**.
- Mix with **shea butter** for enhanced soothing effects.

Pro Tip: Regular use of castor oil can **fade acne scars and dark spots** over time!

Anti-Aging Properties (Reducing Wrinkles and Fine Lines)

Castor oil is a **natural anti-aging powerhouse**, thanks to its ability to **boost collagen and elastin production**. These proteins keep the skin **firm, smooth, and youthful**, reducing **wrinkles, fine lines, and sagging**.

Why Castor Oil is Great for Anti-Aging:

✅ **Deeply Hydrates** – Prevents dryness that makes wrinkles more visible.

✅ **Stimulates Collagen & Elastin** – Keeps skin plump and firm.

✅ **Reduces Free Radical Damage** – Its antioxidants slow down signs of aging.

◆ How to Use for Wrinkles & Fine Lines:

- Dab a small amount of castor oil around **the eyes, forehead, and mouth** before bed.
- Massage in **circular motions** to boost blood flow and absorption.
- Mix with **rosehip oil or vitamin E** for added anti-aging benefits.

Pro Tip: Use **cold-pressed castor oil** for the most potent anti-aging effects!

Treating Scars, Stretch Marks, and Blemishes

Castor oil is well known for its ability to **heal scars, lighten blemishes, and fade stretch marks**. Its **fatty acids penetrate deeply**, promoting **skin cell regeneration and elasticity**.

How Castor Oil Helps with Skin Imperfections:

✅ **Reduces Scars & Blemishes** – Speeds up healing of **cuts, burns, and acne scars.**

✅ **Fades Stretch Marks** – Improves **skin elasticity**, making stretch marks less noticeable.

✅ **Lightens Hyperpigmentation** – Reduces **dark spots and uneven skin tone**.

◆ **How to Use for Scars & Stretch Marks:**

- Gently massage **warm castor oil** onto scars and stretch marks **twice daily**.
- Mix with **aloe vera or coconut oil** for enhanced healing.
- Apply consistently for **4-6 weeks** to see visible results.

Pro Tip: Use castor oil **during pregnancy** to keep the skin hydrated and prevent stretch marks!

DIY Face Masks and Skin Treatments

You can easily create **homemade face masks and skin treatments** with castor oil to **treat acne, brighten skin, and hydrate deeply**.

1. Hydrating Face Mask for Dry Skin

✔ 1 tbsp **castor oil**

✔ 1 tbsp **honey**

✔ ½ mashed **avocado**

How to Use:

Mix all ingredients, apply to the face, leave for **15-20 minutes**, and rinse.

2. Acne-Fighting Face Mask

✔ 1 tbsp **castor oil**

✔ 1 tsp **turmeric powder**

✔ 1 tbsp **yogurt**

How to Use:

Apply to affected areas, leave for **10-15 minutes**, and rinse.

3. Anti-Aging Night Serum

✔ 2 tbsp **castor oil**

✔ 1 tbsp **rosehip oil**

✔ 3 drops **frankincense essential oil**

How to Use:

Massage into the skin before bed for **firm, youthful skin**.

Pro Tip: Use a warm towel to **steam open your pores** before applying castor oil for deeper penetration!

Castor Oil for Hair and Scalp Health

Castor oil is one of the most powerful **natural hair treatments**, known for its ability to **stimulate hair growth, strengthen strands, and improve scalp health**. Whether you're dealing with **hair loss, dandruff, or brittle hair**, castor oil can help restore shine, thickness, and strength.

This chapter explores **how castor oil benefits hair**, the best ways to use it, and simple **DIY hair treatments** for maximum results.

Stimulating Hair Growth and Preventing Hair Loss

One of the most well-known benefits of castor oil is its ability to **promote hair growth**. The high concentration of **ricinoleic acid and omega-6 fatty acids** increases blood circulation to the scalp, nourishing hair follicles and stimulating **faster, thicker hair growth**.

How Castor Oil Helps with Hair Growth:

✅ **Increases Circulation** – More blood flow to hair follicles means **faster, healthier growth**.

✅ **Nourishes Hair Follicles** – Provides essential nutrients like **vitamin E, proteins, and fatty acids**.

✅ **Prevents Hair Thinning & Bald Spots** – Strengthens roots and reduces **shedding**.

◆ **How to Use:**

- Massage **warm castor oil** onto the scalp **2-3 times per week** to stimulate growth.
- Leave it on for **at least 30 minutes or overnight** before washing with a mild shampoo.
- Mix with **peppermint or rosemary essential oil** for added scalp stimulation.

Pro Tip: Use castor oil on eyebrows and eyelashes to boost growth in sparse areas!

Treating Dandruff and Dry Scalp Issues

Castor oil has **antibacterial and antifungal** properties, making it highly effective for treating **dandruff, itchy scalp, and flakiness**. Its deep moisturizing abilities help **soothe scalp irritation and restore balance**.

How Castor Oil Helps with Scalp Health:

✅ **Kills Fungal Growth** – Fights dandruff caused by **yeast or bacterial infections**.

✅ **Hydrates the Scalp** – Prevents **dryness and itchiness**.

✅ **Reduces Scalp Inflammation** – Soothes **redness and irritation**.

🔹 **How to Use for Dandruff & Dry Scalp:**

- Mix **1 tbsp castor oil with 1 tbsp coconut oil** and massage into the scalp.

- Leave it on for **30-60 minutes** before washing.
- Repeat **twice a week** for best results.

Pro Tip: Add a few drops of **tea tree oil** for extra **antifungal power**!

Strengthening Hair Strands and Preventing Breakage

Weak, brittle hair is prone to **split ends and breakage**, leading to slow hair growth. Castor oil **nourishes each strand**, strengthening hair from **root to tip**.

How Castor Oil Strengthens Hair:

✅ **Seals in Moisture** – Prevents hair from becoming **dry and brittle**.

✅ **Coats and Protects Strands** – Creates a protective barrier **against heat and damage**.

✅ **Boosts Keratin Production** – Improves **hair thickness and elasticity**.

🔹 **How to Use for Stronger Hair:**

- Apply **a few drops of castor oil to the ends of your hair** to prevent split ends.
- Use castor oil as a **pre-shampoo treatment** to reduce damage.
- Mix with **argan oil or aloe vera** for added strength and shine.

Pro Tip: Avoid applying too much—castor oil is thick and can make hair feel greasy!

Using Jamaican Black Castor Oil for Maximum Benefits

Jamaican Black Castor Oil (JBCO) is a **more potent version** of regular castor oil. It's made by **roasting castor beans**, which enhances its nutrient profile and makes it even more effective for hair growth.

Benefits of Jamaican Black Castor Oil:

✅ **Higher pH Levels** – Helps **clarify the scalp** and remove buildup.

✅ **More Ricinoleic Acid** – Increases **hair growth stimulation**.

✅ **Stronger Moisturizing Power** – Perfect for **thicker, coarser hair types**.

❖ How to Use Jamaican Black Castor Oil:

- Apply to **edges, bald spots, or thinning areas** to encourage regrowth.
- Mix with **olive oil or shea butter** for deeper penetration.
- Use as a **hot oil treatment** by warming the oil before application.

Pro Tip: JBCO works best for **curly, dry, or thick hair**, while **cold-pressed castor oil** is ideal for **fine or straight hair**!

DIY Hair Masks and Growth Serums

You can make **simple, effective hair treatments** at home using castor oil and natural ingredients.

1. Castor Oil Hair Growth Serum

✓ 2 tbsp **castor oil**

✓ 1 tbsp **argan oil**

✓ 3 drops **rosemary essential oil**

How to Use:

- Mix ingredients in a small bottle.
- Apply a few drops to the **scalp and massage**.
- Use **2-3 times per week** for stronger, healthier hair.

2. Deep Conditioning Hair Mask

✓ 2 tbsp **castor oil**

✓ 1 tbsp **honey**

✓ 1 egg yolk

How to Use:

- Mix ingredients and apply to damp hair.
- Leave for **30-45 minutes**, then rinse with shampoo.
- Use **once a week** for softer, shinier hair.

3. Anti-Dandruff Scalp Treatment

✓ 1 tbsp **castor oil**

✓ 1 tbsp **coconut oil**

✓ 3 drops **tea tree oil**

How to Use:

- Massage into the scalp, leave for **20-30 minutes**, and rinse.
- Use **twice a week** for best results.

Pro Tip: Apply castor oil treatments **before bed** and wash out in the morning for deeper penetration!

Castor Oil for Eye and Oral Health

Castor oil is not only beneficial for **skin and hair** but also plays an important role in **eye and oral health**. With its **deeply hydrating, anti-inflammatory, and antimicrobial properties**, castor oil can help with **dark circles, dry eyes, oral detoxification, and lip care**.

This chapter explores **how castor oil can naturally improve eye health and oral hygiene**, along with step-by-step guides on how to use it safely and effectively.

Reducing Dark Circles and Puffy Eyes

Dark circles and puffy eyes are common problems caused by **lack of sleep, stress, poor circulation, and dehydration**. Castor oil's **anti-inflammatory and moisturizing properties** help reduce puffiness and lighten dark circles over time.

How Castor Oil Helps with Dark Circles:

✅ **Boosts Circulation** – Reduces **fluid retention** under the eyes.

✅ **Deeply Hydrates** – Prevents **dry, sagging skin** around the eyes.

✅ **Rich in Antioxidants** – Helps **fade dark pigmentation** naturally.

◆ **How to Use for Dark Circles & Puffiness:**

1. **Before bed**, take **a small drop of castor oil** on your fingertip.
2. Gently **massage** under your eyes using circular motions.
3. Leave it on overnight and wash your face in the morning.
4. Repeat **daily** for best results.

💡 **Pro Tip:** Mix castor oil with **sweet almond oil or vitamin E** for faster results!

Treating Dry Eyes and Improving Vision Naturally

Castor oil is widely used as a **natural eye lubricant** for people suffering from **dry eyes, irritation, and strain from excessive screen time**.

Some believe it can also **improve vision over time** by reducing inflammation and nourishing the eyes.

How Castor Oil Benefits the Eyes:

✅ **Lubricates Dry Eyes** – Works as a **natural eye drop** alternative.

✅ **Reduces Eye Redness & Irritation** – Soothes **tired, overworked eyes**.

✅ **May Support Vision Health** – Helps **reduce oxidative stress** in the eyes.

🔹 **How to Use for Dry Eyes & Vision Support:**

- Use **cold-pressed, hexane-free castor oil** (MUST be 100% pure).

- **With clean hands**, take a small drop and apply **around the eyelids** before bed.
- **For dry eyes**, some people use a sterile dropper to apply **one drop directly into each eye** (consult a healthcare professional before doing this).
- Blink a few times to spread the oil naturally over the eye surface.

Pro Tip: Use **castor oil eye masks** (cotton pads soaked in castor oil) for 10 minutes to reduce **eye strain and fatigue**!

Oil Pulling with Castor Oil for Oral Detox

Oil pulling is an ancient Ayurvedic practice that involves **swishing oil in the mouth to detoxify the**

body and improve oral health. While coconut and sesame oil are commonly used, castor oil offers **strong antibacterial and antifungal properties** that make it an excellent option for oral detoxification.

Benefits of Oil Pulling with Castor Oil:

✅ **Removes Toxins & Bacteria** – Helps eliminate harmful bacteria from the mouth.

✅ **Improves Gum Health** – Reduces **swelling, bleeding, and inflammation**.

✅ **Whitens Teeth Naturally** – Removes stains and **freshens breath**.

◆ How to Do Oil Pulling with Castor Oil:

1. Take **1 tablespoon** of cold-pressed castor oil.
2. Swish it around in your mouth for **10-20 minutes** (DO NOT swallow).
3. Spit it out into a tissue or trash can (**not the sink** to avoid clogging).
4. Rinse your mouth with **warm water and brush your teeth** as usual.
5. Repeat **3-5 times per week** for best results.

Pro Tip: Add **a drop of peppermint essential oil** for a **fresh taste and added antibacterial benefits!**

Healing Chapped Lips and Mouth Ulcers

Castor oil is **deeply moisturizing** and can **heal cracked, dry lips**, making them soft and supple. It also has **antibacterial and wound-healing properties**, making it effective for treating **mouth ulcers and sores**.

How Castor Oil Helps with Lip & Oral Health:

✅ **Soothes Dry, Chapped Lips** – Locks in moisture and **prevents peeling**.

✅ **Heals Mouth Ulcers** – Speeds up healing and **reduces pain**.

✅ **Protects Against Infections** – Creates a barrier against bacteria.

❖ How to Use for Chapped Lips:

- Apply a drop of castor oil **directly on the lips** before bed.
- Mix with **beeswax and coconut oil** for an all-natural lip balm.
- Use **daily** to keep lips soft and hydrated.

❖ How to Use for Mouth Ulcers:

- Dab a **small amount of castor oil on the sore** using a clean cotton swab.
- Let it sit for **10-15 minutes**, then rinse with warm water.
- Repeat **twice daily** until the ulcer heals.

Pro Tip: Mix castor oil with **honey** for extra healing power on cracked lips or mouth sores!

Castor Oil for Joint and Muscle Pain

Castor oil is widely known for its **anti-inflammatory and pain-relieving properties**, making it an excellent natural remedy for **arthritis, joint pain, muscle soreness, and sports injuries**. Thanks to its high concentration of **ricinoleic acid**, castor oil can penetrate deep into tissues, helping to **reduce inflammation, ease stiffness, and promote healing**.

This chapter explores **how castor oil can be used for pain relief, how to make a castor oil pack, and how it benefits sore muscles and injuries**.

Using Castor Oil for Arthritis and Joint Pain Relief

Arthritis is a condition that causes **joint inflammation, stiffness, and pain**, often affecting the knees, hands, and other weight-bearing joints. Castor oil's **anti-inflammatory and lubricating properties** make it an effective natural treatment for **arthritis, rheumatoid arthritis (RA), and osteoarthritis (OA)**.

How Castor Oil Helps with Joint Pain:

✅ **Reduces Inflammation** – Rich in **ricinoleic acid**, which has natural **anti-inflammatory effects**.

✅ **Improves Joint Mobility** – Helps lubricate stiff joints and **reduces swelling**.

✅ **Provides Deep Pain Relief** – Absorbs into the skin, **soothing aching joints and muscles**.

◆ **How to Use for Arthritis & Joint Pain Relief:**

1. **Warm up** 1-2 tablespoons of castor oil.
2. Massage directly onto **painful joints** in **circular motions** for 5-10 minutes.
3. Cover with a warm towel or heating pad for **better absorption**.
4. Repeat **daily** or **at least 3 times a week** for relief.

Pro Tip: Mix castor oil with **ginger or turmeric essential oil** for enhanced **anti-inflammatory benefits!**

How to Make and Use a Castor Oil Pack for Pain Management

A **castor oil pack** is one of the most effective ways to relieve **chronic pain, inflammation, and muscle soreness**. The heat from the pack allows the castor oil to **penetrate deep into the tissues**, improving **circulation, reducing stiffness, and promoting healing**.

Benefits of Castor Oil Packs for Pain Relief:

✅ **Soothes Aching Joints & Muscles** – Works like a natural **painkiller**.

✅ **Detoxifies and Improves Circulation** – Helps **reduce inflammation** and **remove toxins**.

✅ **Speeds Up Healing** – Great for treating **injuries, swelling, and chronic pain**.

◆ How to Make a Castor Oil Pack:

✓ Materials Needed:

- Organic, cold-pressed castor oil
- A soft, clean **cotton cloth or flannel**
- Plastic wrap or a **waterproof covering**
- A **heating pad or warm towel**

✓ Steps to Use:

1. **Soak the cloth** in warm castor oil (enough to be damp but not dripping).
2. Place the cloth **over the painful area** (joints, muscles, lower back, etc.).
3. Cover with plastic wrap to **keep the oil from spreading**.

4. Apply a heating pad or warm towel **for 30-45 minutes**.
5. Remove the pack and wipe off excess oil.

Pro Tip: Use **3-4 times a week** for **chronic pain** or as needed for muscle soreness!

Treating Sports Injuries and Muscle Soreness

Athletes and active individuals often experience **muscle pain, cramps, and injuries** due to **overuse, strain, or impact**. Castor oil's ability to **increase blood flow, reduce inflammation, and relieve muscle stiffness** makes it a great natural alternative to pain relievers.

How Castor Oil Helps with Muscle Recovery:

✅ **Relaxes Tight Muscles** – Reduces **cramping and muscle fatigue**.

✅ **Speeds Up Healing of Injuries** – Helps treat **sprains, bruises, and minor tears**.

✅ **Prevents Stiffness** – Improves **flexibility and mobility** after workouts.

🔹 **How to Use for Sore Muscles & Sports Injuries:**

- Massage **warm castor oil** onto sore muscles after workouts.
- Apply a **castor oil pack** to injured areas **for 30 minutes** to reduce swelling.

- Mix with **Epsom salt and warm water** for a relaxing **muscle soak**.

Pro Tip: Add a few drops of **peppermint or eucalyptus oil** for an extra **cooling and soothing effect!**

Castor Oil and Women's Health

Castor oil has been used for centuries as a natural remedy for various **women's health concerns**, including **menstrual health, fertility, pregnancy, and postpartum recovery**. With its **anti-inflammatory, circulation-boosting, and hormone-balancing properties**, castor oil is a gentle yet effective solution for many common reproductive health issues.

This chapter explores **how castor oil can help regulate menstrual cycles, improve fertility, support pregnancy recovery, and manage**

conditions like fibroids, PCOS, and ovarian cysts.

Balancing Menstrual Cycles and Reducing PMS Symptoms

Many women experience **irregular periods, painful cramps, bloating, and mood swings** due to **hormonal imbalances and inflammation**. Castor oil can help by **stimulating circulation, reducing inflammation, and promoting natural detoxification of the reproductive organs**.

How Castor Oil Helps with Menstrual Health:

✅ **Reduces Menstrual Cramps** – Soothes **uterine muscles** and relieves tension.

✅ **Regulates Irregular Periods** – Supports **hormonal balance and detoxification**.

✅ **Eases PMS Symptoms** – Reduces **bloating, headaches, and mood swings**.

🔹 **How to Use Castor Oil for Menstrual Relief:**

1. Massage warm castor oil **over the lower abdomen** before or during your period.
2. Use a **castor oil pack** (explained later) **a few days before menstruation** to promote a smoother cycle.
3. Add **lavender or clary sage essential oil** for extra pain relief and relaxation.

Pro Tip: Castor oil packs work best **when used consistently for 3-4 cycles** to see improvements in period regularity and pain relief!

Fertility and Castor Oil (Enhancing Reproductive Health)

For women trying to conceive, castor oil can **support reproductive health by improving circulation, reducing inflammation, and detoxifying the uterus and ovaries**. It's often used in **natural fertility treatments** to help improve conditions that may affect conception.

How Castor Oil Supports Fertility:

✅ **Boosts Blood Flow to the Uterus** – Increases oxygen and nutrient supply to the reproductive organs.

✅ **Supports Hormonal Balance** – Helps regulate estrogen and progesterone levels.

✅ **Aids Detoxification** – Removes toxins from the reproductive system.

🔷 **How to Use Castor Oil for Fertility:**

- Apply a **castor oil pack to the lower abdomen** 3-4 times a week (EXCEPT during menstruation).
- Combine with **a healthy diet, stress reduction, and lifestyle changes** for best results.
- Consult a holistic practitioner if using alongside fertility treatments.

Pro Tip: Avoid castor oil packs **after ovulation if trying to conceive**—use only during the first half of your cycle (before ovulation).

Supporting Pregnancy and Postpartum Healing

During pregnancy and after childbirth, castor oil can be a **gentle, natural support for skin elasticity, pain relief, and postpartum recovery**. However, **castor oil should NOT be ingested during pregnancy unless under medical supervision**, as it can stimulate uterine contractions.

How Castor Oil Helps During Pregnancy & Postpartum:

✅ **Prevents Stretch Marks** – Deeply moisturizes and **improves skin elasticity**.

✅ **Relieves Pregnancy-Related Aches** – Soothes **back pain, swollen feet, and leg cramps**.

✅ **Supports Postpartum Healing** – Helps **heal perineal tears and cesarean scars**.

◆ **Safe Ways to Use Castor Oil in Pregnancy:**

- **For Stretch Marks:** Apply castor oil **on the belly, hips, and thighs** daily.
- **For Pain Relief:** Gently massage on **swollen feet, back, or sore joints**.
- **For Postpartum Healing:** Apply **a few drops on perineal tears or scars** to promote faster healing.

Warning: Avoid ingesting castor oil during pregnancy unless directed by a doctor. It has been used **to induce labor**, but this should only be done under medical supervision!

Castor Oil Packs for Fibroids, PCOS, and Cysts

Fibroids, **polycystic ovary syndrome (PCOS), and ovarian cysts** are common reproductive health conditions that can cause **pain, irregular periods, and hormonal imbalances**. Castor oil packs can help by **improving lymphatic drainage, reducing inflammation, and promoting hormonal balance**.

How Castor Oil Helps with Fibroids, PCOS, and Cysts:

✅ **Reduces Inflammation & Pain** – Helps shrink fibroids and relieve cyst-related discomfort.

✅ **Improves Blood Circulation** – Supports **ovarian and uterine health**.

✅ **Aids in Detoxification** – Helps clear excess **hormones and toxins** from the reproductive system.

◆ **How to Use a Castor Oil Pack for Reproductive Health:**

1. Soak a **cotton cloth or flannel** in warm castor oil.
2. Place over the **lower abdomen**.

3. Cover with **plastic wrap** and apply a **heating pad** for 30-45 minutes.
4. Use **3-4 times a week** for best results (EXCEPT during menstruation).

Pro Tip: Pair castor oil packs with **dietary changes, herbal teas, and stress management** for maximum benefits!

Castor Oil for Detox and Internal Healing

Castor oil has long been used as a powerful natural remedy for **internal detoxification and healing**. Thanks to its **antibacterial, antiviral, and anti-inflammatory properties**, castor oil can help **cleanse the liver, eliminate toxins, remove parasites, and support digestive health**.

This chapter will explore how **castor oil can be used to detox the liver, cleanse the intestines, remove parasites, and support full-body detoxification** while ensuring safe and responsible use.

Liver Cleansing and Detoxification

The **liver** is the body's primary detoxification organ, responsible for **filtering toxins, breaking down hormones, and metabolizing nutrients**. When the liver becomes overloaded with toxins from **processed foods, medications, alcohol, or environmental pollutants**, it can lead to **fatigue, digestive issues, skin problems, and hormonal imbalances**.

How Castor Oil Supports Liver Detox:

✅ **Improves Liver Function** – Enhances the body's ability to remove toxins.

✅ **Stimulates Bile Flow** – Helps break down fats and improve digestion.

✅ **Reduces Inflammation** – Eases liver swelling and improves metabolic processes.

◆ **How to Use a Castor Oil Pack for Liver Detox:**

1. Soak a soft **cotton cloth or flannel** in warm castor oil.
2. Place it over the **right side of the abdomen (over the liver area)**.
3. Cover with **plastic wrap** and apply a **heating pad** for **45–60 minutes**.
4. Relax and allow the oil to penetrate deeply into the liver tissues.
5. Repeat **3-4 times a week** for best results.

Pro Tip: For enhanced detox effects, drink **warm lemon water** or **dandelion tea** after using a castor oil pack!

Using Castor Oil for Parasite Removal

Intestinal parasites can cause **digestive issues, bloating, fatigue, skin problems, and even nutrient deficiencies**. Castor oil works as a natural **anti-parasitic remedy** by helping to **flush out harmful worms and pathogens** from the digestive tract.

How Castor Oil Helps Remove Parasites:

✅ **Stimulates Intestinal Movement** – Expels parasites through bowel movements.

✅ **Kills Harmful Pathogens** – Ricinoleic acid has **antibacterial and antifungal properties**.

✅ **Supports Gut Health** – Helps heal the intestines after parasite removal.

🔹 **How to Use Castor Oil for Parasite Cleansing (Safe Method):**

1. **Take 1 teaspoon of cold-pressed castor oil** mixed with warm water or herbal tea **before bed**.
2. Drink **a glass of warm water with lemon** the next morning to help flush out toxins.
3. Repeat **for 3-5 days only** and then take a break.

4. Combine with **anti-parasitic herbs** like **clove, wormwood, or black walnut** for better results.

Warning: Avoid excessive use, as castor oil has a **strong laxative effect**. Always consult a healthcare professional before using castor oil for internal parasite cleansing!

Castor Oil as a Natural Laxative (Safety Precautions)

One of the most well-known uses of castor oil is as a **natural laxative**. It works by **stimulating bowel movements** and cleansing the intestines. However, it should be used **with caution** to prevent dehydration or dependency.

How Castor Oil Works as a Laxative:

✅ **Stimulates the Bowels** – Increases muscle contractions in the intestines.

✅ **Relieves Occasional Constipation** – Helps empty the bowels naturally.

✅ **Supports Colon Detoxification** – Removes toxins and waste buildup.

🔹 **How to Use Castor Oil for Constipation Relief (Safe Dosage):**

- **Adults:** Take **1-2 teaspoons** on an empty stomach with warm water or juice.

- **Children (over 6 years old):** Use **½ teaspoon** mixed with honey or warm herbal tea.
- Expect a bowel movement **within 4-6 hours**.

Safety Precautions:

❌ Do NOT use castor oil as a laxative **regularly**—only for short-term relief.

❌ Avoid during **pregnancy, breastfeeding, or if you have digestive disorders** like IBS.

❌ Stay **hydrated** to prevent dehydration after taking castor oil.

Full-Body Detox with Castor Oil

Beyond just liver cleansing and digestive health, castor oil can be used for **a complete detox of the body**, helping to **flush out toxins, improve circulation, and boost immunity**.

Benefits of a Full-Body Castor Oil Detox:

✅ **Supports Lymphatic Drainage** – Helps remove toxins from the body.

✅ **Boosts the Immune System** – Strengthens the body's natural defense mechanisms.

✅ **Improves Energy Levels** – Helps the body feel **lighter, cleaner, and more refreshed**.

◆ How to Perform a Castor Oil Detox:

- **Use castor oil packs** on the abdomen, liver, and joints **3-4 times a week**.
- **Drink warm herbal teas** (ginger, dandelion, or fennel) to support digestion.
- **Reduce processed foods, alcohol, and sugar** during your detox period.
- **Stay hydrated** with plenty of water and electrolytes.

Pro Tip: Pair your castor oil detox with a **clean diet and gentle movement (like yoga or stretching)** for even better results!

Castor Oil for Babies and Kids

Castor oil is a gentle yet effective natural remedy that has been used for centuries to **soothe common infant and childhood ailments**. With its **anti-inflammatory, antibacterial, and moisturizing properties**, castor oil can help with **colic, constipation, diaper rash, skin irritations, teething pain, and even cough relief**.

This chapter explores **safe and effective ways to use castor oil for babies and kids**, ensuring that parents can provide their little ones with natural, chemical-free care.

Treating Colic and Constipation in Infants

Colic and constipation are common issues in newborns and infants, often causing **discomfort, crying, and disrupted sleep**. Castor oil, when used externally, can help **soothe tummy troubles, relax the digestive muscles, and promote smooth bowel movements**.

How Castor Oil Helps with Colic and Constipation:

✅ **Relaxes Intestinal Muscles** – Eases gas and bloating.

✅ **Stimulates Bowel Movements** – Gently relieves constipation.

✅ **Soothes Stomach Discomfort** – Reduces cramping and digestive distress.

◆ How to Use Castor Oil for Colic and Constipation:

1. Warm a **few drops of castor oil** by rubbing it between your hands.
2. Gently **massage the baby's tummy** in a **clockwise motion** for 5-10 minutes.
3. For constipation, massage around the **navel area** and lower abdomen.
4. Repeat **once daily** until relief is achieved.

Pro Tip: A warm **castor oil tummy massage before bedtime** can help calm colicky babies and improve sleep.

Safety Note: Never give castor oil **orally** to infants or young children, as it has a strong laxative effect.

Healing Diaper Rash and Skin Irritations

Diaper rash, eczema, and other skin irritations can make babies uncomfortable. Castor oil's **deep moisturizing and antibacterial properties** help **soothe irritation, reduce redness, and promote healing**.

How Castor Oil Helps with Skin Conditions:

✅ **Creates a Protective Barrier** – Shields the skin from moisture and irritation.

✅ **Reduces Inflammation and Redness** – Calms rashes and allergic reactions.

✅ **Speeds Up Healing** – Supports natural skin regeneration.

◆ How to Use Castor Oil for Diaper Rash and Skin Irritations:

- **For Diaper Rash:** Apply a **thin layer of castor oil** after each diaper change to keep the skin moisturized and protected.
- **For Eczema or Dry Patches:** Mix castor oil with **coconut oil** and apply **twice daily**.
- **For Minor Cuts and Scrapes:** Dab a small amount on the affected area to promote healing.

Pro Tip: For extra healing power, mix castor oil with **shea butter or aloe vera** for a soothing diaper rash cream!

Castor Oil for Teething Pain and Cough Relief

Teething can be a difficult time for babies, causing **gum pain, irritability, and excessive drooling**. Additionally, young children are often prone to coughs and congestion. Castor oil can provide **natural relief for both teething and respiratory issues**.

How Castor Oil Helps with Teething:

✅ **Reduces Gum Inflammation** – Soothes swollen gums.

✅ **Eases Discomfort** – Provides mild pain relief.

◆ How to Use Castor Oil for Teething Pain:

- Rub a **tiny amount of castor oil** on the baby's gums using a clean finger.
- Mix with **clove oil** (for babies over 1 year old) for extra numbing relief.
- Repeat **2-3 times a day** as needed.

How Castor Oil Helps with Cough Relief:

✅ **Clears Chest Congestion** – Acts as a natural decongestant.

✅ **Eases Breathing** – Opens airways and relieves coughing.

◆ How to Use Castor Oil for Cough Relief:

1. Warm a few drops of castor oil.

2. Massage it onto the **baby's chest, back, and feet** before bedtime.
3. Add a drop of **eucalyptus or peppermint oil** (for kids over 2 years old) for extra relief.

Pro Tip: Pair a castor oil chest rub with a **warm bath and humidifier** to help your child sleep better during colds!

Castor Oil for Pets and Animals

Castor oil isn't just beneficial for humans—it also provides **natural healing solutions for pets and livestock**. With its **antibacterial, antifungal, anti-inflammatory, and moisturizing properties**, castor oil can be used to **heal wounds, treat skin conditions, and even help with deworming** in animals.

In this chapter, we'll explore **safe and effective ways to use castor oil for dogs, cats, and livestock** while also discussing important precautions to ensure their well-being.

Castor Oil for Wound Healing in Dogs and Cats

Pets are prone to **cuts, scrapes, and minor wounds** from playing outdoors, fighting, or rough surfaces. Castor oil's **natural healing and antimicrobial properties** make it an excellent remedy for **speeding up wound recovery** and preventing infections.

How Castor Oil Helps with Wound Healing:

✅ **Promotes Faster Healing** – Stimulates skin cell regeneration.

✅ **Prevents Infections** – Fights bacteria and fungi that can cause complications.

✅ **Moisturizes the Skin** – Keeps wounds from drying out and cracking.

◆ How to Use Castor Oil for Wound Healing:

1. **Clean the wound thoroughly** with warm water and mild antiseptic soap.
2. Apply **a thin layer of castor oil** directly to the affected area.
3. Cover with a **light bandage** if needed to prevent licking or scratching.
4. Reapply **twice daily** until the wound heals.

Pro Tip: Mix castor oil with **coconut oil or aloe vera** for extra soothing effects!

Caution: Do not use castor oil on **deep wounds, punctures, or surgical stitches** without consulting a veterinarian.

Treating Skin Allergies and Infections in Pets

Many pets suffer from **itchy skin, hot spots, eczema, and fungal infections**. Castor oil's **anti-inflammatory and antimicrobial properties** can help **relieve itching, soothe irritated skin, and eliminate bacterial or fungal infections**.

How Castor Oil Helps with Skin Conditions:

✅ **Relieves Itching and Redness** – Reduces skin irritation caused by allergies.

✅ **Fights Bacterial and Fungal Infections** – Helps treat hot spots, ringworm, and mange.

✅ **Promotes Hair Regrowth** – Stimulates the healing of bald patches from scratching.

❖ How to Use Castor Oil for Skin Allergies and Infections:

- **For Itchy Skin or Hot Spots:** Dab a small amount of castor oil directly on affected areas.
- **For Ringworm or Fungal Infections:** Apply castor oil mixed with a few drops of **tea tree oil** (for dogs only) to fight fungal growth.
- **For Dry Skin or Paw Cracks:** Massage castor oil into the paws or affected areas to provide deep moisture.

Pro Tip: For **large skin infections**, mix castor oil with **apple cider vinegar** and water as a natural spray!

Caution: Avoid using **tea tree oil on cats**, as it can be toxic. Always dilute essential oils before applying to pets.

Natural Deworming Remedy for Livestock and Pets

Parasites can cause serious health issues in pets and farm animals. Castor oil has **mild laxative and anti-parasitic properties**, making it a natural remedy to **help expel worms and intestinal parasites**.

How Castor Oil Helps with Deworming:

✅ **Flushes Out Parasites** – Works as a gentle laxative to remove intestinal worms.

✅ **Supports Digestive Health** – Helps soothe the stomach after parasite removal.

✅ **Enhances Immunity** – Reduces parasite load, improving overall health.

🔹 **How to Use Castor Oil for Natural Deworming (Safe Dosage):**

- **Dogs and Cats:** Mix **½ teaspoon of castor oil** with food once daily for **2-3 days**.

- **Livestock (Goats, Cows, Horses):** Mix **1-2 tablespoons of castor oil** with warm water and administer orally.
- **Poultry (Chickens, Ducks):** Add a few drops of castor oil to feed once a week to help prevent worms.

Pro Tip: Combine castor oil with **pumpkin seeds or black walnut hulls** for a more powerful natural deworming solution!

Caution:

❌ Do NOT give castor oil to **pregnant animals**, as it may cause early labor.

✕ Avoid excessive use—castor oil is a **strong laxative** and should be used **in moderation**.

Castor Oil for Home and Everyday Uses

Castor oil isn't just for health and beauty—it also has a variety of **practical applications around the home**. From **polishing wood furniture and conditioning leather** to **lubricating tools and making homemade beauty products**, castor oil is a versatile and sustainable alternative to chemical-based products.

This chapter explores **how castor oil can be used for household maintenance, DIY projects, and even industrial applications**.

Natural Wood Polish and Leather Conditioner

Over time, wooden furniture and leather goods **lose their shine and develop cracks** due to dryness.

Castor oil acts as a **natural conditioner**, restoring **moisture, shine, and flexibility** while also **protecting against wear and tear**.

How Castor Oil Benefits Wood and Leather:

✅ **Moisturizes and Protects** – Prevents cracking and drying.

✅ **Restores Shine** – Brings back the natural luster.

✅ **Adds a Protective Layer** – Helps repel dust and minor spills.

◆ **How to Use Castor Oil for Wood Polish:**

1. Mix **2 tablespoons of castor oil** with **1 tablespoon of lemon juice**.

2. Apply a **thin layer** to wooden surfaces using a soft cloth.
3. Let it sit for **5-10 minutes**, then buff with a dry cloth.

◆ How to Use Castor Oil for Leather Conditioning:

1. Apply a **few drops** of castor oil to a soft cloth.
2. Rub it into **shoes, bags, or furniture** in circular motions.
3. Let it absorb for **a few hours or overnight**.

Pro Tip: For extra conditioning power, mix castor oil with **beeswax** before applying to leather!

Castor Oil for Lubricating Machinery and Tools

Castor oil has long been used as a **natural lubricant** for **household tools, machinery, and even mechanical engines**. Unlike synthetic lubricants, it is **non-toxic and biodegradable**, making it a safer option for home use.

How Castor Oil Works as a Lubricant:

✅ **Reduces Friction** – Helps tools and machines run smoothly.

✅ **Prevents Rust and Corrosion** – Acts as a protective barrier.

✅ **Extends Lifespan** – Keeps tools in good condition for longer.

🔹 **How to Use Castor Oil for Lubrication:**

- **For Hinges and Locks:** Apply a drop of castor oil to noisy door hinges or stiff locks.
- **For Gardening Tools:** Wipe tools with castor oil after cleaning to prevent rust.
- **For Sewing Machines:** Use a small amount to lubricate moving parts.

Pro Tip: Castor oil is especially effective for **lubricating vintage or delicate machinery**, as it is gentler than synthetic oils!

Making Homemade Soap and Beauty Products

Castor oil is a key ingredient in **natural soaps, lip balms, and beauty products** due to its **moisturizing and antibacterial properties**. It helps create a **rich lather in soaps**, making it a popular choice for DIY skincare formulations.

Benefits of Castor Oil in Homemade Beauty Products:

✅ **Adds Moisture and Hydration** – Perfect for dry skin and lips.

✅ **Creates a Creamy Lather** – Enhances homemade soap quality.

✅ **Acts as a Natural Preservative** – Extends shelf life of beauty products.

◆ **DIY Castor Oil Soap Recipe:**

Ingredients:

- 1 cup of **castor oil**
- 2 cups of **olive oil**

- 1 cup of **coconut oil**
- 1 cup of **lye (sodium hydroxide)**
- 2 cups of **distilled water**

Instructions:

1. Mix **lye and distilled water** in a heat-safe container (use gloves and a mask).
2. In a separate pot, heat **castor oil, coconut oil, and olive oil** until melted.
3. Slowly add the **lye mixture** to the oils, stirring continuously.
4. Blend with a stick blender until it thickens.

5. Pour into a mold and let sit for **24-48 hours** before cutting.
6. Cure the soap for **4-6 weeks** before use.

Pro Tip: Add **essential oils** like lavender or peppermint for fragrance!

◆ Other DIY Beauty Uses:

- **Lip Balm:** Mix castor oil with **beeswax and shea butter** for a nourishing lip treatment.
- **Massage Oil:** Blend castor oil with **sweet almond oil** for a soothing massage.
- **Makeup Remover:** Use castor oil alone or mixed with **jojoba oil** to remove makeup naturally.

Castor Oil in Industrial and Commercial Applications

Beyond home use, castor oil plays a **major role in industrial production**. Its **unique chemical structure** makes it valuable in **biofuels, lubricants, plastics, and cosmetics**.

How Castor Oil is Used in Industries:

✅ **Biofuel Production** – Used in eco-friendly fuel alternatives.

✅ **Manufacturing Lubricants** – Applied in high-performance machinery.

✅ **Making Eco-Friendly Plastics** – Used in biodegradable materials.

✅ **Cosmetic Industry** – Found in lotions, creams, and hair products.

◆ **Examples of Industrial Uses:**

- **Airplane Lubricants:** Castor oil was historically used in **aviation engines** due to its stability at high temperatures.
- **Automobile Greases:** Some **racing car engines** still use castor oil-based lubricants.
- **Biodegradable Plastics:** Castor oil is a key ingredient in **sustainable plastic alternatives**.

Pro Tip: Many **high-end skincare brands** use castor oil in anti-aging creams—so making your own DIY products can save money!

DIY Castor Oil Recipes and Remedies

Castor oil is a powerful natural ingredient that can be used to **enhance beauty, support health, and provide pain relief** through simple DIY remedies. Whether you're looking for a **hair growth serum, healing face cream, detox pack, or anti-aging solution**, this chapter provides **easy-to-follow recipes** to incorporate castor oil into your daily routine.

Homemade Castor Oil Hair Growth Serum

Castor oil is widely known for its ability to **stimulate hair growth, strengthen hair follicles, and prevent hair loss**. This DIY serum is enriched with **essential oils** to further boost hair health.

Ingredients:

✓ 2 tablespoons **castor oil** (Jamaican black castor oil for extra strength)

✓ 1 tablespoon **coconut oil** (moisturizes and prevents breakage)

✓ 5 drops **rosemary essential oil** (stimulates hair growth)

✓ 5 drops **peppermint essential oil** (improves scalp circulation)

Instructions:

1. Mix all ingredients in a small dropper bottle.
2. Shake well before each use.
3. Apply **a few drops** directly to the scalp and massage for **5-10 minutes**.

4. Leave on **overnight** or for at least **2 hours** before washing.
5. Repeat **2-3 times per week** for best results.

Pro Tip: Warm the oil slightly before applying for better absorption!

Healing Castor Oil Face Cream

This **deeply nourishing** face cream hydrates dry skin, **reduces acne**, and promotes a **healthy glow**. It's perfect for those who want an **all-natural, chemical-free moisturizer**.

Ingredients:

✓ 1 tablespoon **castor oil** (deeply hydrates and soothes skin)

✓ 2 tablespoons **shea butter** (rich in vitamins for skin healing)

✓ 1 tablespoon **jojoba oil** (balances oil production)

✓ 5 drops **lavender essential oil** (calms irritation and redness)

✓ 5 drops **frankincense essential oil** (anti-aging and skin rejuvenation)

Instructions:

1. Melt **shea butter** using a double boiler.
2. Remove from heat and mix in **castor oil and jojoba oil**.
3. Let it cool slightly, then add **essential oils**.
4. Stir well and transfer to a small jar.

5. Apply a **pea-sized amount** to clean skin **morning and night**.

Pro Tip: Store in a cool, dark place to keep fresh for **up to 3 months**.

Detoxifying Castor Oil Pack Recipe

A **castor oil pack** is a natural way to **detoxify the liver, improve digestion, and reduce inflammation**. This method is especially beneficial for those experiencing **bloating, sluggish digestion, or hormonal imbalances**.

Ingredients:

✓ 2 tablespoons **cold-pressed castor oil**

✓ 1 piece **organic cotton flannel** (large enough to cover the abdomen)

✓ 1 plastic wrap or **reusable cloth wrap**

✓ 1 **heating pad** or hot water bottle

Instructions:

1. Soak the **cotton flannel** in castor oil until fully saturated.
2. Place the flannel over the **abdomen or lower back** (where detox is needed).
3. Cover with **plastic wrap or a cloth towel** to prevent oil stains.
4. Place a **heating pad** on top and relax for **45-60 minutes**.
5. Remove the pack and wipe the area clean.
6. Repeat **3-4 times per week** for best results.

Pro Tip: Drink **warm lemon water** after using the pack to enhance detoxification.

Castor Oil Massage Blend for Pain Relief

This **warming massage oil** is perfect for **soothing sore muscles, reducing joint pain, and relieving inflammation**. The blend of essential oils enhances **circulation and relaxation**.

Ingredients:

✓ 2 tablespoons **castor oil** (deeply penetrates muscles and joints)

✓ 1 tablespoon **olive oil** (adds extra lubrication)

✓ 5 drops **ginger essential oil** (reduces inflammation)

✓ 5 drops **eucalyptus essential oil** (relieves muscle tension)

✓ 5 drops **black pepper essential oil** (warms and soothes pain)

Instructions:

1. Mix all ingredients in a small glass bottle.
2. Shake well before use.
3. Massage into **sore muscles and joints** for **5-10 minutes**.
4. Apply **daily or as needed** for pain relief.

Pro Tip: For extra relief, cover the massaged area with a **warm towel** to allow deeper absorption.

Anti-Aging Castor Oil Eye Serum

Castor oil is known for its **anti-aging properties**, making it an excellent ingredient for **reducing wrinkles, fine lines, and dark circles** around the eyes. This serum hydrates and plumps the delicate **under-eye area**.

Ingredients:

✓ 1 tablespoon **castor oil** (hydrates and boosts collagen)

✓ 1 teaspoon **sweet almond oil** (lightweight and fast-absorbing)

✓ 5 drops **vitamin E oil** (protects skin and fights free radicals)

✓ 3 drops **rosehip oil** (reduces wrinkles and brightens skin)

Instructions:

1. Combine all ingredients in a **small glass bottle with a dropper**.
2. Shake well before each use.
3. Apply **1-2 drops** under each eye before bed, using your **ring finger** to gently tap the oil into the skin.

Pro Tip: Store in the refrigerator for a **cooling effect** to reduce puffiness!

Conclusion

As we reach the end of this comprehensive guide on **castor oil and its incredible benefits**, it's clear that this ancient remedy continues to be **a powerful tool for health, beauty, and wellness**. From **traditional medicine to modern applications**, castor oil has proven itself as a **versatile and natural solution** for a wide range of concerns.

The Future of Castor Oil in Medicine and Wellness

With the **growing demand for natural and holistic remedies**, castor oil is gaining recognition in **mainstream medicine, alternative health practices, and beauty industries**. Research continues to explore its **anti-inflammatory, antimicrobial, and detoxifying properties**, with studies suggesting its potential role in:

✓ **Chronic Pain Management** – Castor oil packs may help relieve conditions like **arthritis, fibromyalgia, and muscle inflammation**.

✓ **Gut Health and Detoxification** – Its ability to **stimulate lymphatic drainage and remove toxins** makes it a promising remedy for **gut disorders, liver support, and parasite cleansing**.

✓ **Skincare and Anti-Aging** – With its rich fatty acid composition, castor oil is being incorporated into **high-end beauty formulations** for **hydration, anti-aging, and scar healing**.

✓ **Natural Fertility Support** – Many holistic practitioners continue to recommend castor oil packs for **reproductive health, hormone balance, and menstrual regulation**.

✓ **Sustainable and Eco-Friendly Uses** – Castor oil is being used in **biodegradable lubricants, industrial applications, and eco-friendly beauty products**, making it a **sustainable alternative** to synthetic chemicals.

The future of castor oil is **bright**, and as more research emerges, we can expect **new applications in medicine, skincare, and holistic health**.

Final Thoughts and Recommendations

Whether you're using castor oil for **beauty, pain relief, detoxification, or pet care**, the key to success is **consistency and proper application**. To maximize benefits:

✅ **Choose high-quality, cold-pressed castor oil** – This ensures the oil retains its **nutrients and healing properties**.

✅ **Perform a patch test** before applying to large areas of skin to **avoid potential irritation**.

✅ **Use regularly for best results** – Hair growth, skin healing, and pain relief require **ongoing**

application for noticeable improvements.

✅ **Store in a cool, dark place** to maintain its **freshness and potency**.

✅ **Experiment with different DIY recipes** to find what works best for **your specific needs**.

Incorporating castor oil into your routine can lead to **amazing transformations** in your **health and well-being**. The more you explore its **versatility**, the more you'll discover its **endless benefits**!

Where to Buy High-Quality Castor Oil

To get the **most benefits** from castor oil, it's important to **choose the right product**. Here's what to look for when purchasing:

🛒 **Cold-Pressed and Hexane-Free** – Avoid chemically processed oils, as they **lose beneficial nutrients**.

🛒 **100% Pure and Organic** – Ensure it's **free from additives, preservatives, or synthetic ingredients**.

🛒 **Glass Bottle Packaging** – Helps **preserve the oil** better than plastic, reducing contamination.

Recommended Sources for Buying Castor Oil:

✓ **Health Food Stores** – Many local organic stores carry high-quality castor oil.

✓ **Online Retailers** – Websites like **Amazon, iHerb, Thrive Market, and Mountain Rose Herbs** offer a variety of trusted brands.

✓ **Specialty Natural Beauty Shops** – Stores specializing in **organic and Ayurvedic products** often sell **premium-quality castor oil**.

Pro Tip: Read reviews and check for **third-party certifications** to ensure **purity and authenticity**!

Frequently Asked Questions (FAQs)

This section addresses **common concerns and misconceptions** about castor oil, helping readers **use it safely and effectively**.

1. Can I drink castor oil for detox?

Yes, but with caution! **Castor oil is a powerful laxative**, so it should only be taken **in small doses (1 teaspoon max) and not for extended periods**. Overuse can lead to dehydration and electrolyte imbalances. Always consult a healthcare provider before internal use.

2. How long does it take for castor oil to work?

The results depend on the **application and the condition being treated**:

✓ **Hair Growth** – Visible changes in **4-8 weeks** with regular use.

✓ **Pain Relief** – Relief can be felt **within 30-60 minutes** of applying a castor oil pack.

✓ **Skin Healing** – Acne and scars may improve in **1-3 weeks**.

✓ **Laxative Effect** – Typically works within **6-8 hours** of ingestion.

3. Is castor oil safe for pregnant women?

Externally, castor oil is **safe** and can be used for **stretch marks and skin hydration**. However, **taking castor oil orally is NOT recommended** during pregnancy unless under medical supervision, as it may **induce labor**.

4. Can I use castor oil on my pets?

Yes! Castor oil can be used for **minor wounds, skin infections, and parasite control** in pets. However, **avoid oral consumption**, as it may cause digestive issues in some animals. Always consult a veterinarian before using it internally.

5. Will castor oil clog my pores?

No! Castor oil is **non-comedogenic** (low on the pore-clogging scale) and is safe for most skin types. It has **natural antibacterial properties** that help with acne rather than causing breakouts. If you have oily skin, **mix it with lighter oils like jojoba or grapeseed oil**.

6. How often should I use castor oil for hair growth?

For best results, apply castor oil **2-3 times a week** to the scalp and massage thoroughly. Using too much oil too often can lead to **product buildup**, so wash it out properly after application.

7. What is the best type of castor oil for hair and skin?

✓ **Jamaican Black Castor Oil (JBCO)** – Best for **thicker hair growth and scalp health**.

✓ **Cold-Pressed Castor Oil** – Ideal for **sensitive skin, acne, and anti-aging**.

✓ **Hydrogenated Castor Oil (Castor Wax)** – Used in **cosmetics and industrial applications** but not recommended for skin/hair.

8. Can castor oil be used on eyebrows and eyelashes?

Absolutely! Apply **a small amount** to eyebrows and lashes using **a clean spoolie brush or cotton swab** before bed. Results can be seen in **4-6 weeks** with consistent use.

www.ingramcontent.com/pod-product-compliance
Lightning Source LLC
LaVergne TN
LVHW050915210926
848482LV00012B/450
* 9 7 9 8 3 4 8 5 8 5 2 2 8 *